KEGEL EXERCISE FOR MEN AND WOMAN

HOW TO PERFORM KEGEL FOR BOTH MEN AND WOMEN AND THEIR BENEFITS

WARDEN REYNOLDS

Table of Contents

CHAPTER ONE

KEGEL EXERCISE FOR MEN AND WOMAN

Both men and women can benefit from KEGEL EXERCISE!

Kegel Exercises: What Are They?

Strengthening your pelvic floor muscles through kegel exercises is a common goal. Pelvic floor exercises are another name for them. Muscles that support your uterus, urinary bladder, small intestine, and rectum are affected by the medication. In addition to helping you stay in shape, kegels can help you avoid bladder leaks and accidental bowel movements. They can even enhance the quality of your sex.

In-Depth Knowledge on the Kegel Exercise

When your pelvic floor muscles are working as they should, you may not even think about them. Your body's natural defenses become less effective as you get older. Pelvic organ prolapse is a medical term for this condition (POP). Essentially, the organs in your pelvis begin to droop. It is possible for them to enter or exit your vagina. After a hysterectomy, your vaginal tissues may begin to protrude from your body.

POP can also be brought on by the following factors:

- Pregnancy

- Giving birth vaginally.

Surgery in the pelvic region is an option (C-section or hysterectomy)

• Genetics

Coughing, laughing, or sneezing frequently (it pushes on the pelvic organs)

Kegel exercises are not just for women. Additionally, they have the ability to strengthen the muscles in the male pelvic floor as well. Your bladder and bowels are supported by these muscles, as well as your sex life. Doing kegels can help if you suffer from incontinence, such as dribbling when you pee. A better orgasm and better control over ejaculation can be achieved through the use of these products.

For both men and women:
Kegel exercises

People of all ages can benefit from kegel exercises, which strengthen the muscles of the pelvic floor. For both males and females, here is some basic information to get you started with Kegel exercises.

Exercising the Pelvic Floor

Female reproductive organs are supported by the pelvic floor muscles, which include the rectum, small intestine, bladder and uterus, respectively. Pregnancy, childbirth, surgery, and old age can all weaken the muscles. Having weak Kegel muscles can lead to incontinence. Kegel exercises should be performed on a regular basis in order to prevent or improve the strength of these muscles.

CHAPTER TWO

Determine the muscles of the pelvic floor before beginning a kegel exercise. To find these muscles, simply stop urinating in the middle of a swab. Identifying the right muscles will allow you to perform these exercises at any time.

Each session should include five seconds of contraction and relaxation of the muscles in your pelvic floor. Intervals can be increased to 10 seconds as you become more physically fit. Do at least three sets of 10 repetitions of Kegel exercises each day to get the best results.

Exercising the Kegel Muscles

Men can benefit from these as well, despite the fact that they are typically associated with women's health. Enhance your bladder control by doing kegel exercises. In addition, they may help with the treatment of prostatitis, and they can improve your sex drive. Many men have found that performing Kegel exercises on a regular basis helps prevent premature ejaculation. Conclusion

To begin a Kegel exercise, locate the muscles that need to be worked. Stopping the flow of urine before your bladder is completely empty will help you locate these muscles The first step is to identify the muscles you want to work on.

As a rule of thumb, novices should contract and relax these muscles three to five times per minute. It is possible to extend these intervals, however, as you get stronger. Kegel exercises should be performed at least three times a day. Each set should have a minimum of ten repetitions.

Other Factors to Consider

When performing Kegel exercises, men and women alike should be careful not to overextend their muscles. Relaxed buttocks, thighs, and abdominal muscles yield the best results. Exercise while urinating can increase the risk of a urinary tract infection in both men and women.

Exercises for the Kegel Muscles

Try to go to the bathroom and see if you can relieve yourself. Squeeze your muscles as soon as the urine begins to flow to keep it contained. A tightening of the muscles is normal. The muscles that keep you from passing gas can be squeaky clean by squeezing them. You've only done one Kegel so far. Relax the muscle, then repeat the process.

But don't get into the habit of doing Kegels while you're going to the bathroom. Other issues, such as urinary tract infections, may arise as a result of this.

Start out slowly. Squeeze and release your pelvic floor muscles three times in quick succession. Repeat this process ten times. That's the first one. Try to do as many as you can at first, and then work your way up to 10. Two or three times a day, perform one set of 10 Kegels.

They are not harmful. As a matter of fact, you can incorporate them into your daily schedule. During the time you're brushing your teeth or driving, eating dinner, or watching television, do these exercises.

Doctor's Appointments

If you're having trouble performing Kegels, seek assistance. It's best to ask your doctor for advice on how to carry out these tasks. There are also helpful tools, such as:

- Cones in the vagina. These weights can be inserted into the vagina and held in place by contractions of the pelvic muscles.

- Biofeedback. Both men and women will be fitted with a pressure sensor by your doctor. A monitor tracks the movement of your pelvic floor muscles as you contract and relax them.

The Benefits of Kegel Exercise

Within a few weeks or months, the majority of women who

perform Kegels on a regular basis notice a reduction in urine leakage. Your doctor can help you if you're still concerned about a prolapse or don't feel your symptoms are getting better.

CHAPTER THREE

Perils of the Kegel

Even though kegels are safe, caution should always be exercised. Here's what you need to look for:

Avoid doing Kegel exercises while you pee. Instead of actually stopping yourself from peeing, you're supposed to tense your muscles as if you were. The risk of developing a urinary tract infection is possible (UTI).

• Don't go overboard with your workouts. It's possible that this will cause you to strain when you go to the bathroom.

• Make it a point to stay active on a regular basis. Kegels, like other exercises, benefit from repetition and consistency if you want to improve your strength. For at least 15 weeks, you'll need to do these exercises daily. Consult your physician before making any alterations to your daily routine.

Some people aren't a good fit for kegel exercises. You may be doing more harm than good by performing these exercises if your muscles in the pelvic floor are always tight. Muscles that are already fatigued will not be able to respond if you try to contract them. Find out if this applies to you by consulting with your doctor about the possibility of it.

What are the names of the muscles in my pelvic floor?

The pelvic floor muscles run from your pubic bone in the

front of your body to your tailbone (the back end of your spine) in the back, forming a small'sling or hammock.'

It's easy to locate the muscles of your pelvic floor. When you're sitting on the toilet, try to stop the flow of your urine. Only do this once you've gotten used to the sensation (otherwise this stopping and starting of urine flow can lead to other health problems). Alternatively, you can use your vaginal muscles to squeeze a finger inserted into your vagina. You should be able to feel a slight tenseness around your fingertip at this point. When you do Kegel exercises, you build the same muscles that feel like they're 'lifting' inside you when you try these activities.

How do I perform Kegel exercises?

Lifting, holding, and then relaxing your pelvic floor muscles is how you perform Kegel exercises. In the beginning, focus on a small number of exercises (such as lifting and stretching) for a short period of time, and then gradually increase the duration of each'session' as well as the variety and number of exercises performed (which is called a set). Perform two sets of each exercise every day.

Lifting and holding for three seconds, followed by three seconds of relaxation, is a good place to start. Make sure you do this 10 times in succession, and you'll have completed one set. To begin with, if 10 times in a row is too much, decrease this number.) Make a point to perform these exercises at least twice per day. All of these numbers should be increased as you get better. That is to say, increase the number of repetitions, the amount of time spent lifting and holding each exercise, and the number of times per day you perform these exercises. Rather than holding for three seconds and relaxing for three seconds, hold for four seconds and relax for up to five seconds. Aim to complete a set of 10 exercises in a row (if not already there). Finally, up the frequency of your workouts from twice daily to three daily.

CHAPTER FOUR

Kegel exercises can be improved using biofeedback training and electric stimulation of the pelvic floor muscles. It is possible to use electrical stimulation to simulate the sensation of a properly performed Kegel exercise through the use of biofeedback.

A health care professional inserts a biofeedback training

probe into the vagina. A monitor checks to see if the correct muscles are being squeezed when someone is performing a Kegel exercise.

An electric current is applied to the muscles of the pelvic floor via electrical stimulation. These muscles tense up as a result. This feeling is similar to what you should get from performing a Kegel exercise correctly.

Exercises for the kegel

While sitting or standing, you can perform Kegel exercises.

Starting with laying down exercises can help if your pelvic muscles are weak. Exercise should begin with a few minutes of exercise in the morning and at night.

• Do only as many Kegel exercises as are comfortable for you to begin with (eg, five Kegels for three seconds each twice a day). As you gain strength and endurance, gradually increase these numbers.

• Breathe out while doing the exercises – don't hold your

breath. Also, avoid squeezing or bearing down on your inner thighs, back, buttocks, or stomach muscles while exercising. You're not doing the exercise correctly if you're squeezing these muscles.

Equipment for "Kegel muscle strengthening" is not required. Even though it may be beneficial, some equipment may not be as effective as advertised.

When should I begin to notice a difference?

Women who begin and maintain a Kegel exercise regimen report less urine leakage within 12 weeks.

It's not just women who benefit from Kegel exercises.

It's a matter of fact. Kegel exercises can also be beneficial for men with certain health and sexual health issues. These exercises in men can:

• Assist with incontinence management (depending on the cause).

Treatment of prostatitis and benign prostatic hyperplasia-related pain and swelling in the prostate (BPH).

• Improve orgasm sensation and ejaculatory control in men to increase their sexual pleasure.

THE END